You Might Need To LOSE WEIGHT

NOTE: This book is not intended to make fun of anyone. Excess weight can lead to serious health issues. If you feel you need to lose a few extra pounds or more, MAJIK weight loss pills may be a good solution to help you on that journey. Please take care of your body. Consider giving MAJIK a try. Get back to the person who shared this with you for more details and samples.

Compiled by
Nick Hetcher

Laughter

Is

Good

Medicine

Proverbs 17:22

You Might Need To LOSE WEIGHT

You Might Need To LOSE WEIGHT...   if your shadow weighs more than you do.

You Might Need To LOSE WEIGHT... if your belly button has its own zip code.

You Might Need To LOSE WEIGHT... if you've become a frequent flyer at all-you-can-eat buffets.

You Might Need To LOSE WEIGHT... if your treadmill files for divorce due to neglect.

You Might Need To LOSE WEIGHT... if you can't fit through a revolving door without a can of WD-40.

You Might Need To LOSE WEIGHT... if your nickname is "Snack Attack."

You Might Need To LOSE WEIGHT... if your doctor prescribes donuts for depression.

You Might Need To LOSE WEIGHT... if you have to call a moving company to roll you out of bed.

You Might Need To LOSE WEIGHT... if your self-esteem is on a temporary vacation.

You Might Need To LOSE WEIGHT... if your sweatpants have stretch marks.

You Might Need To LOSE WEIGHT... if you're considering hiring a personal trainer, for your pet hamster.

You Might Need To LOSE WEIGHT... if you have a designated driver just to help you get off the couch.

You Might Need To LOSE WEIGHT... if your jeans have their own gravitational pull.

You Might Need To LOSE WEIGHT... if your cereal bowl requires a building permit.

You Might Need To LOSE WEIGHT... if your yoga instructor suggests you try sumo wrestling instead.

You Might Need To LOSE WEIGHT... if your favorite exercise is lifting the TV remote.

You Might Need To LOSE WEIGHT... if your diet plan includes "Netflix and Pizza."

You Might Need To LOSE WEIGHT... if you've named your love handles "Bacon" and "Bits."

You Might Need To LOSE WEIGHT... if your salad dressing is considered a condiment bath.

You Might Need To LOSE WEIGHT... if you can't remember the last time you saw your toes.

You Might Need To LOSE WEIGHT... if your belly button is an innie and an outie at the same time.

You Might Need To LOSE WEIGHT... if your doctor refers to you as a "walking food court."

You Might Need To LOSE WEIGHT... if your food pyramid has pizza as the foundation.

You Might Need To LOSE WEIGHT... if you confuse burpees with "blurpees" because you can't see while doing them.

You Might Need To LOSE WEIGHT... if your bathroom scale switches to scientific notation when you step on it.

You Might Need To LOSE WEIGHT... if your favorite exercise is lifting bags of chips to your mouth.

You Might Need To LOSE WEIGHT... if you've mastered the art of inhaling snacks without chewing.

You Might Need To LOSE WEIGHT... if your favorite diet is

the "see-food" diet – you see food and you eat it.

You Might Need To LOSE WEIGHT... if you've invented a dance move called "the food coma."

You Might Need To LOSE WEIGHT... if your belly button has its own Facebook page with more friends than you.

You Might Need To LOSE WEIGHT... if your personal trainer quit and opened a bakery instead.

You Might Need To LOSE WEIGHT... if you've been told you have a "way with buffets."

You Might Need To LOSE WEIGHT... if your refrigerator has more magnets than a science lab.

You Might Need To LOSE WEIGHT... if you have a black belt in ordering takeout.

You Might Need To LOSE WEIGHT... if your food cravings have their own fan club.

You Might Need To LOSE WEIGHT... if your refrigerator door has its own revolving entry system.

You Might Need To LOSE WEIGHT... if your dance moves are inspired by the wobble of jelly.

You Might Need To LOSE WEIGHT... if your favorite exercise is "recliner push-ups" — pushing yourself up from the couch.

You Might Need To LOSE WEIGHT... if your grocery list is longer than the aisle itself.

You Might Need To LOSE WEIGHT... if your Fitbit sends you condolence cards for being inactive.

You Might Need To LOSE WEIGHT... if your gym membership comes with a free meal plan.

You Might Need To LOSE WEIGHT... if you need a separate closet just for your stretchy pants.

You Might Need To LOSE WEIGHT... if your favorite exercise is "heavy breathing" – it's a real calorie burner!

You Might Need To LOSE WEIGHT... if you've mastered the art of eating while sleeping.

You Might Need To LOSE WEIGHT... if your doctor refers to you as a "muffin-top model."

You Might Need To LOSE WEIGHT... if your idea of a marathon is a "marathon of snacks."

You Might Need To LOSE WEIGHT... if your personal motto is "will work for cake."

You Might Need To LOSE WEIGHT... if you've been offered sponsorship deals with most fast food chains.

You Might Need To LOSE WEIGHT... if your favorite exercise is "scrolling" – on social media, not the treadmill.

You Might Need To LOSE WEIGHT... if you can't remember

the last time you saw your toes without bending over.

You Might Need To LOSE WEIGHT... if your doctor suggests you try a "seated workout" – preferably in front of the TV.

You Might Need To LOSE WEIGHT... if you require a crane to lift you out of bed in the morning.

You Might Need To LOSE WEIGHT... if your favorite exercise is "mindless munching" –

burning calories while day dreaming about food.

You Might Need To LOSE WEIGHT... if your reflection in the mirror shouts, "Incoming!"

You Might Need To LOSE WEIGHT... if you've been mistaken for a sumo wrestler during a costume party.

You Might Need To LOSE WEIGHT... if your idea of a warm-up is microwaving a slice of pizza.

You Might Need To LOSE WEIGHT... if your body fat percentage has its own zip code.

You Might Need To LOSE WEIGHT... if your favorite exercise is "exercising your right to eat."

You Might Need To LOSE WEIGHT... if your motivation to exercise needs a forklift.

You Might Need To LOSE WEIGHT... if your pantry has more snacks than a convenience store.

You Might Need To LOSE WEIGHT... if your waistline has its own time zone.

You Might Need To LOSE WEIGHT... if your idea of a "cheat day" is every day of the week.

You Might Need To LOSE WEIGHT... if your favorite exercise is "food speed-eating" – breaking records, not calories.

You Might Need To LOSE WEIGHT... if your personal

trainer has become a certified donut connoisseur.

You Might Need To LOSE WEIGHT... if your favorite workout attire is elastic waistbands and stretchy socks.

You Might Need To LOSE WEIGHT... if your scale gives up and starts using scientific notation.

You Might Need To LOSE WEIGHT... if your favorite exercise is "exercising your right to eat whatever and wherever you want."

You Might Need To LOSE WEIGHT... if you need a forklift to find your motivation to exercise.

You Might Need To LOSE WEIGHT... if your favorite exercise is "plate spinning" – keeping multiple dishes filled with food, in the air all at the same time.

You Might Need To LOSE WEIGHT... if your idea of "meal prep" is ordering takeout in advance.

You Might Need To LOSE WEIGHT... if your calorie counting app crashes due to overload.

You Might Need To LOSE WEIGHT... if your favorite workout is lifting a pint of ice cream to your mouth.

You Might Need To LOSE WEIGHT... if your gym towel doubles as a bib.

You Might Need To LOSE WEIGHT... if your treadmill is

covered in more dust than a museum exhibit.

You Might Need To LOSE WEIGHT... if your favorite workout equipment is the TV remote and a bag of chips.

You Might Need To LOSE WEIGHT... if your idea of a "cleanse" is switching from regular soda to diet soda.

You Might Need To LOSE WEIGHT... if your exercise routine consists of reaching for the TV remote and doing finger curls.

You Might Need To LOSE WEIGHT... if your favorite snack is "air" because you can eat a lot of it.

You Might Need To LOSE WEIGHT... if your gym bag has more snacks than workout gear.

You Might Need To LOSE WEIGHT... if your workout playlist consists solely of songs about food.

You Might Need To LOSE WEIGHT... if your idea of portion

control is eating pizza one slice at a time.

You Might Need To LOSE WEIGHT... if your favorite exercise is "chewing gum lifting" – the only resistance training you do.

You Might Need To LOSE WEIGHT... if your fitness goals involve reaching the end of a bag of chips.

You Might Need To LOSE WEIGHT... if your favorite workout move is the "nap and curl" – napping with a dumbbell in hand.

You Might Need To LOSE WEIGHT... if your love for food is stronger than your willpower to lose weight.

You Might Need To LOSE WEIGHT... if your scale sends you hate mail.

You Might Need To LOSE WEIGHT... if your idea of portion control is cutting a pizza into four slices instead of eight.

You Might Need To LOSE WEIGHT... if your favorite fitness gadget is a remote control with extra-long reach.

You Might Need To LOSE WEIGHT... if your workout playlist is a compilation of chewing sounds.

You Might Need To LOSE WEIGHT... if your refrigerator door has more fingerprints than a crime scene.

You Might Need To LOSE WEIGHT... if your treadmill has become a clothes hanger.

You Might Need To LOSE WEIGHT... if your idea of a "workout buddy" is your food delivery person.

You Might Need To LOSE WEIGHT... if your favorite exercise is "carb lifting" – bringing a donut to your mouth.

You Might Need To LOSE WEIGHT... if your favorite

fitness class is "nap-robics" – exercising while snoozing.

You Might Need To LOSE WEIGHT... if your grocery cart has its own VIP section for special snacks.

You Might Need To LOSE WEIGHT... if your step counter resets itself at midnight out of sympathy.

You Might Need To LOSE WEIGHT... if your favorite exercise is "chair yoga" – sitting and pretending to stretch.

You Might Need To LOSE WEIGHT... if your cheat day is longer than the other six days of the week. In fact it last 3 days.

You Might Need To LOSE WEIGHT... if your favorite workout equipment is a TV tray for snacks.

You Might Need To LOSE WEIGHT... if your idea of a "healthy smoothie" is a chocalate milkshake with a blueberry.

You Might Need To LOSE WEIGHT... if your meal plan

consists solely of different flavors of potato chips.

You Might Need To LOSE WEIGHT... if your favorite exercise is "doughnut dodging" – avoiding temptation in the bakery aisle.

You Might Need To LOSE WEIGHT... if you consider a sugar rush to be your preferred form of cardio.

You Might Need To LOSE WEIGHT... if your idea of portion

control is eating a spoonful of sugar with each meal.

You Might Need To LOSE WEIGHT... if your fitness routine involves doing jumping jacks in a field of cotton candy.

You Might Need To LOSE WEIGHT... if your snack cravings are solely focused on sugary treats that can rival Willy Wonka's Factory.

You Might Need To LOSE WEIGHT... if your workout playlist is a compilation of songs that make you want to dance with a sugar spoon.

You Might Need To LOSE WEIGHT... if your gym bag is filled with packets of sugar instead of weights or exercise gear.

You Might Need To LOSE WEIGHT... if your motivation to exercise is the promise of a post-workout dessert buffet.

You Might Need To LOSE WEIGHT... if your favorite exercise is "caramel caramelizing"

– perfecting the art of making caramel at home.

You Might Need To LOSE WEIGHT... if your meal plan revolves around finding creative ways to incorporate sugar into every dish.

You Might Need To LOSE WEIGHT... if your fitness goals involve mastering the art of eating sugar while minimizing tooth decay.

You Might Need To LOSE WEIGHT... if your gym

membership card is primarily used to enter candy shops and confectioneries, after hours.

You Might Need To LOSE WEIGHT... if your favorite exercise is "marshmallow tossing" – tossing marshmallows into your mouth from a distance.

You Might Need To LOSE WEIGHT... if your workout routine includes "lollipop lunges" – lunging forward to grab lollipops with your mouth.

You Might Need To LOSE WEIGHT... if your idea of calorie counting is estimating the sugar content of everything you eat.

You Might Need To LOSE WEIGHT... if your favorite workout is "gummy bear squats" – squatting down to pick up gummy bears from the floor.

You Might Need To LOSE WEIGHT... if your snack stash is exclusively filled with sugary delights that could put a candy shop to shame.

You Might Need To LOSE WEIGHT... if your exercise routine consists of skipping rope made of licorice. Then eating it as your reward.

You Might Need To LOSE WEIGHT... if your workout playlist is a mix of sugary pop songs that keep you moving and craving more sweets.

You Might Need To LOSE WEIGHT... if your gym bag is filled with chocolate bars and candy wrappers instead of workout essentials.

You Might Need To LOSE WEIGHT... if your motivation to exercise is the thought of earning a sugar-filled reward afterward.

You Might Need To LOSE WEIGHT... if your favorite exercise is "cotton candy twirling" – spinning cotton candy into fluffy perfection.

You Might Need To LOSE WEIGHT... if your fitness routine involves "jelly bean juggling" – tossing jelly beans in the air and catching them in your mouth.

You Might Need To LOSE WEIGHT... if your snack drawer is a treasure trove of sugary delights that would make any dentist cringe.

You Might Need To LOSE WEIGHT... if your workout attire features sugary prints and patterns to showcase your sweet tooth.

You Might Need To LOSE WEIGHT... if your idea of portion control is eating sugar cubes by the handful.

You Might Need To LOSE WEIGHT... if your exercise routine consists of chasing the ice cream truck down the street.

You Might Need To LOSE WEIGHT... if your favorite workout is "candy cane curls" – curling candy canes instead of dumbbells.

You Might Need To LOSE WEIGHT... if your refrigerator is stocked with containers of different flavored sugars instead of fresh produce.

You Might Need To LOSE WEIGHT... if your fitness goals involve finding innovative ways to incorporate sugar into every meal.

You Might Need To LOSE WEIGHT... if your favorite exercise is "sprinkles tossing" – sprinkling colorful sugar sprinkles onto your favorite treats.

You Might Need To LOSE WEIGHT... if your snack stash is filled with candy bars, chocolate kisses, and sugar-coated delights.

You Might Need To LOSE WEIGHT... if your workout playlist is a collection of catchy tunes that make you crave candy.

You Might Need To LOSE WEIGHT... if your gym bag is a secret sugar stash disguised as a regular gym bag.

You Might Need To LOSE WEIGHT... if your motivation to exercise is the promise of indulging in a sugar-filled feast afterward.

You Might Need To LOSE WEIGHT... if your gym membership card hasn't been used in so long it's expired.

You Might Need To LOSE WEIGHT... if your favorite exercise is "elevator surfing" – taking the elevator to go up one floor.

You Might Need To LOSE WEIGHT... if your idea of a "full-body workout" is stretching to reach the snack shelf.

You Might Need To LOSE WEIGHT... if your favorite way to hydrate is with a 6-pack.

You Might Need To LOSE WEIGHT... if your weight loss strategy involves changing your middle name to "Salad."

You Might Need To LOSE WEIGHT... if your meal prep involves ordering takeout from different restaurants.

You Might Need To LOSE WEIGHT... if your treadmill is a perfect spot for hanging laundry.

You Might Need To LOSE WEIGHT... if your favorite exercise is "texting thumbs" – building finger muscles while scrolling.

You Might Need To LOSE WEIGHT... if your favorite sport is competitive snacking.

You Might Need To LOSE WEIGHT... if your motivation to work out is the promise of a post-workout milkshake.

You Might Need To LOSE WEIGHT... if your workout

clothes have never seen a drop of sweat.

You Might Need To LOSE WEIGHT... if your idea of "meal prepping" is ordering from the drive-thru in advance.

You Might Need To LOSE WEIGHT... if your favorite exercise is "remote control weightlifting" – changing channels is your workout.

You Might Need To LOSE WEIGHT... if your gym bag is

mainly used for storing snacks and soda.

You Might Need To LOSE WEIGHT... if your favorite workout is lifting a spoon to your mouth as many times as possible in 10 minutes.

You Might Need To LOSE WEIGHT... if your idea of portion control is using a bigger plate.

You Might Need To LOSE WEIGHT... if your fridge has a "snack zone" and a "real food zone."

You Might Need To LOSE WEIGHT... if your gym visits are just for your Instagram photos.

You Might Need To LOSE WEIGHT... if your favorite workout move is the "snooze button press."

You Might Need To LOSE WEIGHT... if your idea of a "home workout" is changing the channel without using the remote.

You Might Need To LOSE WEIGHT... if your favorite

fitness equipment is a bag of chips for resistance training.

You Might Need To LOSE WEIGHT... if your motivation to exercise is imagining the dessert waiting for you.

You Might Need To LOSE WEIGHT... if your gym membership card doubles as a pizza coupon.

You Might Need To LOSE WEIGHT... if your favorite exercise is "guilt-free snacking" – pretending calories don't count.

You Might Need To LOSE WEIGHT... if your fitness routine involves practicing your "hover hand" while reaching for treats.

You Might Need To LOSE WEIGHT... if your idea of "healthy fats" is eating an entire jar of peanut butter.

You Might Need To LOSE WEIGHT... if your favorite exercise is "bed-to-fridge sprints" – racing for snacks in the morning.

You Might Need To LOSE WEIGHT... if your water bottle is always filled with soda.

You Might Need To LOSE WEIGHT... if your fitness goals involve being able to eat more without gaining weight.

You Might Need To LOSE WEIGHT... if your favorite exercise is "cupcake curls" – lifting cupcakes to your mouth.

You Might Need To LOSE WEIGHT... if your motivation to

work out is the promise of a post-workout dessert buffet.

You Might Need To LOSE WEIGHT... if your workout routine consists of binge-watching your favorite TV shows.

You Might Need To LOSE WEIGHT... if your favorite fitness equipment is a bag of potato chips for finger exercises.

You Might Need To LOSE WEIGHT... if your idea of portion control is eating pizza with a larger fork.

You Might Need To LOSE WEIGHT... if your gym bag is filled with snack wrappers instead of workout gear.

You Might Need To LOSE WEIGHT... if your favorite exercise is "burger flipping" – flipping burgers on the grill.

You Might Need To LOSE WEIGHT... if your exercise routine involves breakdancing with a vacuum cleaner.

You Might Need To LOSE WEIGHT... if your snack cravings

have evolved into a full-blown interpretive dance routine.

You Might Need To LOSE WEIGHT... if your refrigerator has become a portal to a parallel universe filled with low-calorie alternatives.

You Might Need To LOSE WEIGHT... if your favorite workout is "hula-hooping with a flamingo" – combining balance and eccentricity.

You Might Need To LOSE WEIGHT... if your meal plan

includes a daily serving of kale-flavored toothpaste.

You Might Need To LOSE WEIGHT... if your fitness routine consists of doing jumping jacks in zero gravity.

You Might Need To LOSE WEIGHT... if your snack stash is stored inside a hidden compartment in your pet's hamster wheel.

You Might Need To LOSE WEIGHT... if your idea of portion

control is eating soup with a ladle the size of a canoe paddle.

You Might Need To LOSE WEIGHT... if your workout attire includes a cape for extra aerodynamic calorie burning.

You Might Need To LOSE WEIGHT... if your refrigerator speaks to you in motivational quotes every time you open it.

You Might Need To LOSE WEIGHT... if your favorite exercise is "toe-tapping telekinesis" – moving editable objects with the power of your mind and feet.

You Might Need To LOSE WEIGHT... if your snack cravings have reached the level of seeking out rare and exotic fruits from undiscovered islands.

You Might Need To LOSE WEIGHT... if your gym membership comes with a personal trainer who is an actual wizard.

You Might Need To LOSE WEIGHT... if your meal prep

involves carving intricate sculptures out of tofu and broccoli.

You Might Need To LOSE WEIGHT... if your fitness goals include mastering the art of levitating while lying on the sofa.

You Might Need To LOSE WEIGHT... if your snack drawer is a secret doorway to a magical realm of guilt-free indulgence.

You Might Need To LOSE WEIGHT... if your workout playlist is a compilation of catchy tunes performed by singing vegetables.

You Might Need To LOSE WEIGHT... if your refrigerator has a built-in holographic personal chef who offers healthy cooking tutorials.

You Might Need To LOSE WEIGHT... if your favorite exercise is "cloud surfing" – floating through the sky on puffs of fluffy clouds made of marshmallows.

You Might Need To LOSE WEIGHT... if your workout routine includes synchronized swimming in a bathtub filled with rainbow-colored smoothies.

You Might Need To LOSE WEIGHT... if your snack stash is guarded by an imaginary enchanted forest of broccoli trees and carrot bushes.

You Might Need To LOSE WEIGHT... if your fitness regimen includes "extreme spoon-bending" — sculpting spoons into works of art with your mind.

You Might Need To LOSE WEIGHT... if your refrigerator doors automatically lock after sunset to prevent midnight snacking.

You Might Need To LOSE WEIGHT... if your favorite workout is "disco yoga" – stretching and grooving to funky beats in a dazzling light show.

You Might Need To LOSE WEIGHT... if your exercise routine consists of interpretive dance battles against imaginary opponents.

You Might Need To LOSE WEIGHT... if your snack cravings have led you to explore the mystical world of unicorn-approved superfoods.

You Might Need To LOSE WEIGHT... if your gym offers classes in levitation aerobics and anti-gravity weightlifting.

You Might Need To LOSE WEIGHT... if your meal plan involves crafting intricate fruit sculptures that resemble famous landmarks.

You Might Need To LOSE WEIGHT... if your snack drawer magically refills itself with perfectly portioned, calorie-free treats.

You Might Need To LOSE WEIGHT... if your workout playlist features ambient sounds of nature mixed with motivational speeches from wise old trees.

You Might Need To LOSE WEIGHT... if your refrigerator has a built-in teleportation device to instantly transport you to a healthy restaurant of your choice.

You Might Need To LOSE WEIGHT... if your workout routine includes "moonwalking on water" – defying gravity and getting fit with style.

You Might Need To LOSE WEIGHT... if your favorite exercise is "bubble wrap popping" – releasing stress and calories with every satisfying pop.

You Might Need To LOSE WEIGHT... if your snack stash is stored inside a time capsule, ensuring you always have a supply of nostalgic treats.

You Might Need To LOSE WEIGHT... if your idea of portion control involves using a magnifying glass to admire your tiny plate of food.

You Might Need To LOSE WEIGHT... if your fitness regimen includes synchronized trampoline bouncing with a group of acrobatic dolphins.

You Might Need To LOSE WEIGHT... if your refrigerator doors are covered in motivational quotes and inspirational artwork.

You Might Need To LOSE WEIGHT... if your favorite workout is "juggling flaming dumbbells" – a fiery and intense full-body workout.

You Might Need To LOSE WEIGHT... if your workout playlist is composed entirely of food-related songs.

You Might Need To LOSE WEIGHT... if your food cravings have their own social media following.

You Might Need To LOSE WEIGHT... if your fitness goals involve finding ways to exercise while sitting down.

You Might Need To LOSE WEIGHT... if your favorite workout is lifting the remote to change channels.

You Might Need To LOSE WEIGHT... if your idea of a "healthy snack" is a bag of chips with a side of dip.

You Might Need To LOSE WEIGHT... if your fitness routine

consists of doing stretches to reach snacks on the top shelf.

You Might Need To LOSE WEIGHT... if your refrigerator is a treasure trove of leftovers and snacks.

You Might Need To LOSE WEIGHT... if your favorite exercise is "food tasting" – sampling everything in sight.

You Might Need To LOSE WEIGHT... if your workout attire is a collection of stretchy pants and oversized T-shirts.

You Might Need To LOSE WEIGHT... if your idea of calorie tracking is taking mental notes of every dessert you see.

You Might Need To LOSE WEIGHT... if your favorite workout is doing the "snack dash" – running to get snacks during TV commercials.

You Might Need To LOSE WEIGHT... if your fitness motivation comes from envisioning yourself as a professional eater.

You Might Need To LOSE WEIGHT... if your meal prep involves ordering from every restaurant on your street.

You Might Need To LOSE WEIGHT... if your new favorite exercise is "licking the spoon" while baking.

You Might Need To LOSE WEIGHT... if your idea of "portion control" is eating a family-sized meal by yourself.

You Might Need To LOSE WEIGHT... if your fitness routine

is based on finding the quickest way to the nearest snack.

You Might Need To LOSE WEIGHT... if your gym membership card is mainly used to open bags of chips.

You Might Need To LOSE WEIGHT... if your new favorite workout is balancing a plate of food on your lap.

You Might Need To LOSE WEIGHT... if your idea of "carb cycling" is eating a variety of bread products every day.

You Might Need To LOSE WEIGHT... if your workout playlist consists of songs about greasy food and nothing else.

You Might Need To LOSE WEIGHT... if your snack stash is more impressive than a vending machine.

You Might Need To LOSE WEIGHT... if your favorite exercise is "chair dancing" – grooving in your seat while snacking.

You Might Need To LOSE WEIGHT... if your fitness goals involve finding creative ways to incorporate chips into every meal.

You Might Need To LOSE WEIGHT... if your meal plan is based on trying every fast food item on the menu.

You Might Need To LOSE WEIGHT... if your favorite workout is lifting your phone to order takeout.

You Might Need To LOSE WEIGHT... if your idea of

"intermittent fasting" is eating a snack between every meal.

You Might Need To LOSE WEIGHT... if your gym visits are mostly for socializing at the fast food joints on the way there, and on the way home.

You Might Need To LOSE WEIGHT... if your fitness routine involves mastering the art of eating while walking.

You Might Need To LOSE WEIGHT... if your favorite exercise is "sitting up and down" –

getting in and out of chairs repeatedly.

You Might Need To LOSE WEIGHT... if your idea of "meal planning" is figuring out which drive-thru to visit each day.

You Might Need To LOSE WEIGHT... if your favorite workout is lifting your fork to your mouth during mealtime.

You Might Need To LOSE WEIGHT... if your fitness tracker is confused by your lack of movement and excessive snacking.

You Might Need To LOSE WEIGHT... if your grocery list consists mostly of snacks and desserts.

You Might Need To LOSE WEIGHT... if your favorite exercise is "shopping cart sprints" – racing through the grocery store aisles.

You Might Need To LOSE WEIGHT... if your idea of portion

control is eating pizza with a knife and fork.

You Might Need To LOSE WEIGHT... if your fitness routine includes "chair aerobics" – exercising while seated.

You Might Need To LOSE WEIGHT... if your refrigerator is better stocked than the local deli.

You Might Need To LOSE WEIGHT... if your favorite workout is "burrito rolling" – perfecting the art of wrapping.

You Might Need To LOSE WEIGHT... if your gym bag doubles as a snack storage container.

You Might Need To LOSE WEIGHT... if your motivation to exercise involves picturing yourself at an all-you-can-eat buffet.

You Might Need To LOSE WEIGHT... if your favorite exercise is "door-to-fridge lunges" – frequent trips to grab snacks.

You Might Need To LOSE WEIGHT... if your meal plan revolves around finding new dessert recipes.

You Might Need To LOSE WEIGHT... if your idea of a "balanced meal" is a plate with equal portions of pizza and fries.

You Might Need To LOSE WEIGHT... if your fitness routine includes "couch squats" – getting up and down to grab snacks.

You Might Need To LOSE WEIGHT... if your refrigerator door is a collage of takeout menus.

You Might Need To LOSE WEIGHT... if your favorite exercise is "bagel curls" – lifting bagels to your mouth.

You Might Need To LOSE WEIGHT... if your snack drawer has more variety than a college vending machine.

You Might Need To LOSE WEIGHT... if your workout attire

consists of oversized T-shirts to hide the food baby.

You Might Need To LOSE WEIGHT... if your idea of calorie burning is eating spicy food for a temporary metabolism boost.

You Might Need To LOSE WEIGHT... if your favorite workout is "pancake flipping" – perfecting the art of flipping pancakes.

You Might Need To LOSE WEIGHT... if your meal prep

involves planning the next local fast food restaurant to visit.

You Might Need To LOSE WEIGHT... if your fitness routine is mostly comprised of reaching for snacks on and under the couch.

You Might Need To LOSE WEIGHT... if your gym membership card is permanently lost in a pile of snack wrappers.

You Might Need To LOSE WEIGHT... if your favorite exercise is "dishwashing squats" –

bending down to load the dishwasher.

You Might Need To LOSE WEIGHT... if your idea of "protein intake" is eating an entire tub of ice cream in one sitting.

You Might Need To LOSE WEIGHT... if your workout playlist consists of songs that mention food cravings.

You Might Need To LOSE WEIGHT... if your snack stash is hidden in every corner of your home.

You Might Need To LOSE WEIGHT... if your favorite exercise is "fast-food relay" – running to pick up various takeout orders.

You Might Need To LOSE WEIGHT... if your fridge is so packed with food that items always fall out when you open the door.

You Might Need To LOSE WEIGHT... if your fitness goals involve finding new ways to incorporate bacon into every meal.

You Might Need To LOSE WEIGHT... if your meal plan is simply choosing between different flavors of chips.

You Might Need To LOSE WEIGHT... if your favorite workout is "microwave dash" – sprinting to the microwave before the timer goes off.

You Might Need To LOSE WEIGHT... if your exercise routine consists of lifting your fork to your mouth in rapid succession.

You Might Need To LOSE WEIGHT... if your idea of "food pyramid" is a tower of stacked pizza boxes.

You Might Need To LOSE WEIGHT... if your workout playlist is a collection of jingles from fast food commercials.

You Might Need To LOSE WEIGHT... if your snack cravings have become a source of inspiration for local bakeries.

You Might Need To LOSE WEIGHT... if your fitness goals

involve finding the perfect balance between eating and napping.

You Might Need To LOSE WEIGHT... if your idea of portion control is taking two servings of everything.

You Might Need To LOSE WEIGHT... if your gym bag is filled with empty chip bags and soda cans instead of workout gear.

You Might Need To LOSE WEIGHT... if your favorite exercise is "munchie marathons" – snacking while binge-watching.

You Might Need To LOSE WEIGHT... if your refrigerator shelves are organized by snack categories.

You Might Need To LOSE WEIGHT... if your meal prep consists of arranging snacks in colorful containers.

You Might Need To LOSE WEIGHT... if your favorite exercise is "pillow planking" – holding a pillow while lying down.

You Might Need To LOSE WEIGHT... if your idea of a "healthy dessert" is putting fruit on top of a mountain of ice cream.

You Might Need To LOSE WEIGHT... if your fitness routine involves pretending to do push-ups while actually napping.

You Might Need To LOSE WEIGHT... if your refrigerator is a treasure trove of condiments but lacks any real food.

You Might Need To LOSE WEIGHT... if your favorite

workout is "food pyramid balancing" – trying to eat an equal amount from each sugar group.

You Might Need To LOSE WEIGHT... if your workout playlist is an audio recording of someone chewing.

You Might Need To LOSE WEIGHT... if your gym bag is filled with coupons for fast food instead of gym clothes.

You Might Need To LOSE WEIGHT... if your motivation to

exercise is the thought of burning off the calories from a single bite.

You Might Need To LOSE WEIGHT... if your favorite exercise is "pizza stretching" – pulling apart slices of pizza.

You Might Need To LOSE WEIGHT... if your meal plan revolves around finding new ways to incorporate chocolate into every dish.

You Might Need To LOSE WEIGHT... if your idea of "mindful eating" is focusing on how good the food tastes, without considering portion sizes.

You Might Need To LOSE WEIGHT... if your fitness routine includes "couch to fridge" sprints for snack refills.

You Might Need To LOSE WEIGHT... if your refrigerator is like a game of Jenga, with food precariously stacked inside.

You Might Need To LOSE WEIGHT... if your favorite exercise is "burger flipping" –

flipping burgers on the grill with exaggerated movements.

You Might Need To LOSE WEIGHT... if your snack drawer is better organized than your entire kitchen.

You Might Need To LOSE WEIGHT... if your workout attire is primarily designed for maximum stretchability.

You Might Need To LOSE WEIGHT... if your favorite workout is "TV commercial crunches" – doing sit-ups only during commercial breaks.

You Might Need To LOSE WEIGHT... if your meal plan involves ordering every dessert on the menu and calling it a "dessert tasting experience."

You Might Need To LOSE WEIGHT... if your fitness routine includes "grocery shopping speed-walking" – rushing to get to the snack aisle.

You Might Need To LOSE WEIGHT... if your gym

membership card is mostly used to swipe for free samples at the local grocery store.

You Might Need To LOSE WEIGHT... if your favorite exercise is "biscuit curls" – lifting biscuits to your mouth instead of dumbbells.

You Might Need To LOSE WEIGHT... if your snack stash is so vast it could rival a convenience store.

You Might Need To LOSE WEIGHT... if your workout

consists of flexing your imagination while daydreaming about food.

You Might Need To LOSE WEIGHT... if your idea of a "healthy breakfast" is eating a doughnut while sipping a sweet, green smoothie.

You Might Need To LOSE WEIGHT... if your fitness goals revolve around finding ways to exercise without getting out of bed.

You Might Need To LOSE WEIGHT... if your meal prep involves arranging snacks in perfect Instagram-worthy patterns.

You Might Need To LOSE WEIGHT... if your favorite workout is "chocolate truffle squatting" – bending down to pick up fallen truffles.

You Might Need To LOSE WEIGHT... if your exercise routine consists of carrying multiple grocery bags in one trip to save time for more snacking.

You Might Need To LOSE WEIGHT... if your refrigerator door is decorated with magnets advertising your favorite takeout places.

You Might Need To LOSE WEIGHT... if your fitness regimen includes "couch jumping" – leaping from couch to couch during TV marathons.

You Might Need To LOSE WEIGHT... if your idea of "portion control" is eating a slice of cake with a larger fork.

You Might Need To LOSE WEIGHT... if your workout playlist is a compilation of the sound of popcorn popping.

You Might Need To LOSE WEIGHT... if your snack cravings have led you to develop a new language solely based on different chip flavors.

You Might Need To LOSE WEIGHT... if your fitness goals involve finding creative ways to eat while lying down.

You Might Need To LOSE WEIGHT... if your meal plan revolves around trying every limited-edition flavor of your favorite snacks.

You Might Need To LOSE WEIGHT... if your favorite exercise is "kettle chip swinging" – swinging a bag of kettle chips like a kettlebell.

You Might Need To LOSE WEIGHT... if your workout routine consists of shadowboxing while holding a slice of pizza in each hand.

You Might Need To LOSE WEIGHT... if your idea of "balanced eating" is eating a burger with a side of fries in each hand.

You Might Need To LOSE WEIGHT... if your snack cupboard is so full it requires a strategic plan to open without items falling out.

You Might Need To LOSE WEIGHT... if your workout routine involves "chair dancing" while munching on snacks.

You Might Need To LOSE WEIGHT... if your refrigerator shelves are so packed that you need a map to locate anything.

You Might Need To LOSE WEIGHT... if your favorite workout is "donut spinning" — spinning a donut on your finger instead of a basketball.

You Might Need To LOSE WEIGHT... if your exercise routine is simply lifting a slice of pizza to your mouth and calling it a bicep curl.

You Might Need To LOSE WEIGHT... if your snack stash is meticulously organized by flavor, brand, and calorie count.

You Might Need To LOSE WEIGHT... if your workout attire is adorned with food-related slogans and illustrations.

You Might Need To LOSE WEIGHT... if your idea of "calorie-burning" is vigorously shaking a bag of snacks before opening it.

You Might Need To LOSE WEIGHT... if your favorite exercise is "ice cream cone balancing" – seeing how long you can balance an ice cream cone without it toppling.

You Might Need To LOSE WEIGHT... if your meal plan involves trying every new flavor of potato chips that hits the market.

You Might Need To LOSE WEIGHT... if your fitness routine includes "doughnut squats" – squatting down to pick up doughnuts from a box.

You Might Need To LOSE WEIGHT... if your refrigerator is a testament to your love for condiments and sauces.

You Might Need To LOSE WEIGHT... if your favorite workout is "remote control weightlifting" – changing channels is your main source of exercise.

You Might Need To LOSE WEIGHT... if your snack drawer is like a hidden treasure chest full of tasty treats.

You Might Need To LOSE WEIGHT... if your idea of portion control is eating directly from the family-sized snack bag.

You Might Need To LOSE WEIGHT... if your favorite exercise is "cookie dunking" – perfecting the art of dipping cookies in milk.

You Might Need To LOSE WEIGHT... if your workout playlist consists of songs with lyrics that make you crave food.

You Might Need To LOSE WEIGHT... if your favorite exercise is "taco folding" – honing your skills in folding tacos perfectly.

You Might Need To LOSE WEIGHT... if your workout routine involves "TV treadmill walking" – walking on the treadmill while binge-watching your favorite shows.

You Might Need To LOSE WEIGHT... if your idea of calorie burning is vigorously stirring your coffee in the morning.

You Might Need To LOSE WEIGHT... if your favorite workout is "cookie sheet lifting" – lifting cookie sheets loaded with freshly baked treats, without spilling any.

You Might Need To LOSE WEIGHT... if your exercise routine includes "potato chip crunches" – crunching potato chips instead of doing traditional ab exercises.

You Might Need To LOSE WEIGHT... if your meal plan revolves around finding creative ways to make dessert the main course.

You Might Need To LOSE WEIGHT... if your fitness goals involve becoming a professional taste tester.

You Might Need To LOSE WEIGHT... if your gym membership card is mainly used as a bookmark for your favorite recipe.

You Might Need To LOSE WEIGHT... if your favorite exercise is "cookie dough rolling"

– rolling cookie dough into *perfect* balls.

You Might Need To LOSE WEIGHT... if your snack drawer is more organized than your closet.

You Might Need To LOSE WEIGHT... if your workout attire is designed to stretch and accommodate your love for food.

You Might Need To LOSE WEIGHT... if your idea of "meal prep" is ordering takeout from a different restaurant every day of the week.

You Might Need To LOSE WEIGHT... if your fitness routine includes "couch surfing" – switching between shows without getting up.

You Might Need To LOSE WEIGHT... if your refrigerator is a never-ending supply of beverages but lacks any real sustenance.

You Might Need To LOSE WEIGHT... if your favorite

exercise is "candy bar lifting" –
lifting candy bars instead of
dumbbells.

You Might Need To LOSE
WEIGHT... if your snack stash is
strategically hidden from others to
avoid sharing.

You Might Need To LOSE
WEIGHT... if your fitness goals
involve mastering the art of eating
while lying down.

You Might Need To LOSE
WEIGHT... if your meal plan
consists of various ways to

incorporate candy bars into every dish.

You Might Need To LOSE WEIGHT... if your favorite workout is "bagel biting" – biting into bagels with enthusiasm.

You Might Need To LOSE WEIGHT... if your exercise routine involves lifting a spoonful of ice cream to your mouth for resistance training.

You Might Need To LOSE WEIGHT... if your idea of portion

control is eating directly from the chip bag until it's empty.

You Might Need To LOSE WEIGHT... if your gym visits are primarily to take selfies in trendy workout gear.

You Might Need To LOSE WEIGHT... if your favorite exercise is "pretzel twisting" – perfecting the art of twisting pretzels into different shapes.

You Might Need To LOSE WEIGHT... if your workout playlist is a mix of fast-food jingles and catchy snack commercials.

You Might Need To LOSE WEIGHT... if your snack stash is so vast it requires multiple hiding spots throughout the house.

You Might Need To LOSE WEIGHT... if your fitness routine includes "chip bag lunges" – lunging across the room to grab another chip bag.

You Might Need To LOSE WEIGHT... if your refrigerator is

filled with more takeout containers than actual groceries.

You Might Need To LOSE WEIGHT... if your favorite exercise is "soda can curls" – curling soda cans instead of weights.

You Might Need To LOSE WEIGHT... if your workout attire is designed to accommodate maximum food consumption.

You Might Need To LOSE WEIGHT... if your idea of calorie tracking is guessing the calorie count based on the size of the food portion.

You Might Need To LOSE WEIGHT... if your favorite workout is "marshmallow catching" – tossing marshmallows in the air and catching them with your mouth.

You Might Need To LOSE WEIGHT... if your exercise routine consists of walking to the kitchen for frequent snack breaks.

You Might Need To LOSE WEIGHT... if your snack drawer

is like a hidden treasure trove of sugary delights.

You Might Need To LOSE WEIGHT... if your motivation to exercise is the thought of a post-workout feast.

You Might Need To LOSE WEIGHT... if your favorite exercise is "waffle flipping" – flipping waffles in the air while preparing breakfast.

You Might Need To LOSE WEIGHT... if your daily workout involves chasing after the ice cream truck while riding a unicycle.

You Might Need To LOSE WEIGHT... if your refrigerator has a built-in DJ booth that spins funky tunes while you search for healthy snacks.

You Might Need To LOSE WEIGHT... if your meal plan includes a strict regimen of eating with chopsticks made entirely of candy canes.

You Might Need To LOSE WEIGHT... if your fitness routine

involves climbing up the stairs of a skyscraper using a ladder made of licorice.

You Might Need To LOSE WEIGHT... if your snack stash is hidden inside a puzzle box that can only be opened by solving riddles about nutrition.

You Might Need To LOSE WEIGHT... if your idea of portion control is measuring your food by the number of mini marshmallows it would take to cover it.

You Might Need To LOSE WEIGHT... if your refrigerator has a holographic image of a personal trainer who cheers you on during late-night fridge raids.

You Might Need To LOSE WEIGHT... if your idea of portion control is measuring your food by the number of gummy bears that can fit in your palm.

You Might Need To LOSE WEIGHT... if your snack cravings have led you to invent a new language based entirely on the names of different ice cream flavors.

TRY MAJIK...

One capsule designed to change your eating behavior, manage blood sugar, support heart health while providing super focus, elevated mood and all-day energy.

If you'd like to experience the incredible weight loss and wellness benefits of **MAJIK**... make sure to get back to the person who shared this book with you, for more information and samples.

Disclaimer: The information provided on this product label or packaging is for educational purposes only and is not intended to replace professional medical advice or guidance. If you have any specific medical conditions or concerns, please consult with your healthcare provider before using this product.

This product may contain ingredients that may cause sensitivities in some individuals. Please carefully review the ingredients list and discontinue use if you experience any adverse reactions.

Please keep this nutritional product out of reach of children. Do not exceed the recommended dosage or use if the safety seal is broken or missing.

The statements made regarding this product have not been evaluated by the Food and Drug Administration (FDA)]. This product is not intended to diagnose, treat, cure, or prevent any disease.

Other Joke Books by

Nick Hetcher

THE **COFFEE** JOKE BOOK
TheCoffeeJokeBook.com

THE ENCYCLOPEDIA OF **DAD** JOKES DadJokeBook.com

THE ENCYCLOPEDIA OF **CAT** JOKES CatJokeBook.com